Prostate

Benign Prostate Enlargement

Revised and Updated

Gentlemen Discover Information + Solutions

by
John Harriyott

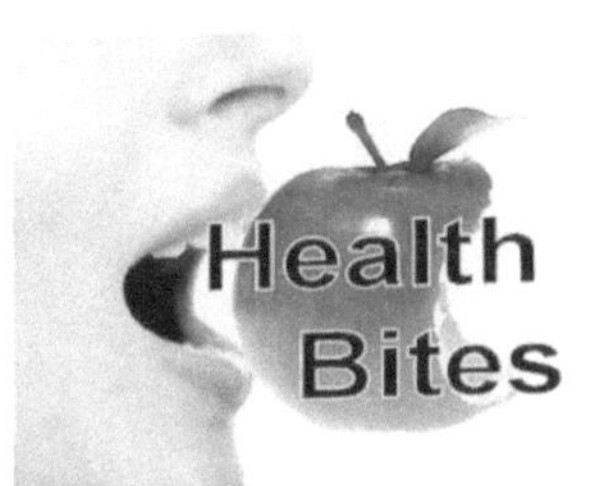

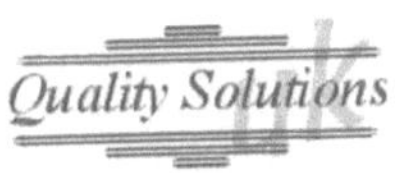

Contents

     Quality Solutions

Introduction

More information, special offers and a wide range of interesting "commodities" can be viewed at quality-solutions.co.uk

Most likely, you don't want to spend a lot of time thinking about your prostate. But if you are finding that you are having issues such as trouble urinating, your prostate may be what's keeping you awake at night.

Around the time of your 45th birthday, your prostate begins to grow. This is called benign prostatic hyperplasia (BPH), a condition that develops slowly and increases as we men get older.

While BPH is not cancer, it is the swelling of your prostate beyond normal size and still requires treatment.

Approximately one-third of men older than 50 have an enlarged prostate. This number increases to 90 percent by age 85. As men, we are slow to recognize the problem and even slower at seeking a solution.

Benign enlargement of the prostate is the more common condition in which your prostate gland swells beyond normal size. If you have this disorder, keep in mind that it is not a cancer, although it still requires treatment.

It is always sensible to check with your doctor to make sure it is benign and not cancerous.

Background

The prostate gland is only found in men and is normally about the size of a walnut. It lies immediately below the bladder and just above the penis. A tube called the urethra, which carries urine from your bladder, passes through the centre of the prostate gland.

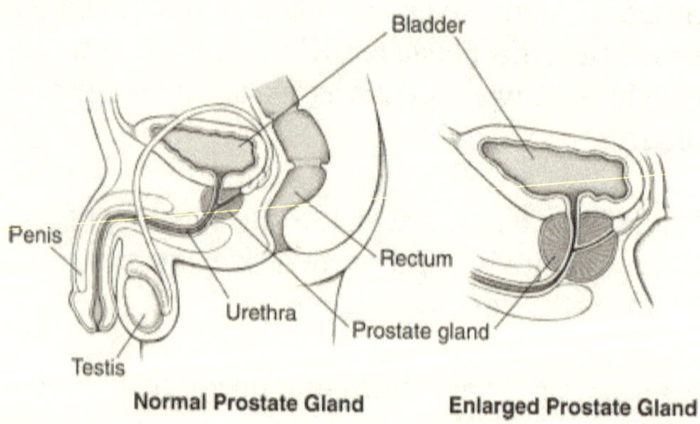

An enlarged prostate can press on the urethra, which causes narrowing or blockage of the tube and prevents your urine from flowing normally.

    Quality Solutions

Symptoms.

If your prostate becomes enlarged, you may experience some of the following symptoms, which tend to worsen as time goes on:

- an increased need to urinate during the night
- finding it difficult to start urinating
- a need to pass urine more often
- urine continues to dribble out after you have finished urinating
- having a flow that is weak
- having a flow that stops and starts
- feeling you have to strain to produce urine
- feeling as if your bladder has not emptied properly

On an average day it is normal to pass urine up to once during the night and four to eight times during the daytime.

Causes

In the early stage of prostate enlargement, the bladder muscle becomes thicker and forces urine through the narrowed urethra by contracting more powerfully.

As a result, the bladder muscle may become more sensitive, causing a need to urinate more often and more suddenly.

The prostate grows larger due to an increase in the number of cells (hyperplasia). However, the precise reason for this increase is unknown.

A variety of factors may be involved, including androgens (male hormones), oestrogens, growth factors and other cell signalling pathways.

Obesity increases the risk of BPH, while exercise can lower your risk.

Having an enlarged prostate doesn't affect your risk of developing prostate cancer.

As the prostate grows larger and the urethra is squeezed more tightly, the bladder might not be able to fully compensate for the problem and completely empty.

Other causes

Whilst not a cause, it is known that obesity increases the risk of BPH. So if you are not yet at an advanced stage of BPH then keeping your weigh under control would be a sensible route to follow.

Similarly Drinking more fluid, up to eight glasses of water per day, may help prevent infection. However, for men already suffering with increased urinary frequency, this may only exacerbate the problem

Solutions

Below are suggestions for **relieving** prostate problems.

Eliminating enlarged prostate is through surgery which is discussed later on.

Stop drinking any liquids for one to two hours before going to bed. This will help to prevent nocturia (waking up during the night to pass urine).

Stop drinking caffeine, these days there is a plentiful supply of decaffeinated coffee and tea.

Reduce or limit your consumption alcohol.

Exercise regularly. Research has shown that moderate exercise, such as walking for 30 to 60 minutes a day, can improve the situation (although it is unclear exactly why this is). These suggestions do ease the problem, providing you make the effort to follow through and do the work suggested.

Supplements

Saw palmetto is an herbal remedy that comes

from a type of palm tree. It's been used in traditional medicine for centuries to relieve urinary symptoms, including those caused by an enlarged prostate.

Pygeum comes from the bark of the African plum tree and has been used in traditional medicine to treat urinary problems since ancient times. It's often used to treat BPH symptoms, especially in Europe.

Nettle root has been found to lessen BPH symptoms, and is widely used in Europe. Sometimes nettle is used in combination with other natural BPH remedies, such as pygeum or saw palmetto.

Rye grass pollen extracts are made from three types of grass pollen—rye, timothy, and corn. This supplement seems to be especially helpful for preventing the need to get up during the night and use the bathroom. It can also help men urinate more completely, so there is less urine left in their bladder afterwards.

Medicines

Alpha blockers, such as tamsulosin (Flomax) and alfuzosin (Uroxatral), silodosin (Rapaflo) relax the muscles in the prostate and thus may relieve symptoms.

Finasteride (Proscar) or dutasteride (Avodart) can cause the prostate to shrink. As a result, the urinary symptoms may improve. These drugs are most helpful in men who have at least moderate enlargement of the prostate.

Tadalafil (Cialis for daily use) has recently been approved for the treatment of BPH.

If you find that they are not working for you, then your condition may be far more serious and another visit to your doctor is recommended.

Surgery

If your prostate does not respond to drug treatment, or if it is quite large, surgery may be necessary to remove the enlarged portion of the gland.

What is involved in prostate surgery?

Prostate surgery is an operation to remove some or most of an enlarged prostate gland so that urine can flow more freely.

Prostate surgery is usually performed under general anaesthesia, which means that you will be asleep during the procedure.

However, for some men, epidural or spinal anaesthesia is preferable. This completely blocks the feeling in your pelvis and legs, but you will still be awake.

Your surgeon and anaesthetist will discuss which type of anaesthesia is most suitable for you.

The most common operation is known as **TURP**, which stands for transurethral resection of the prostate.

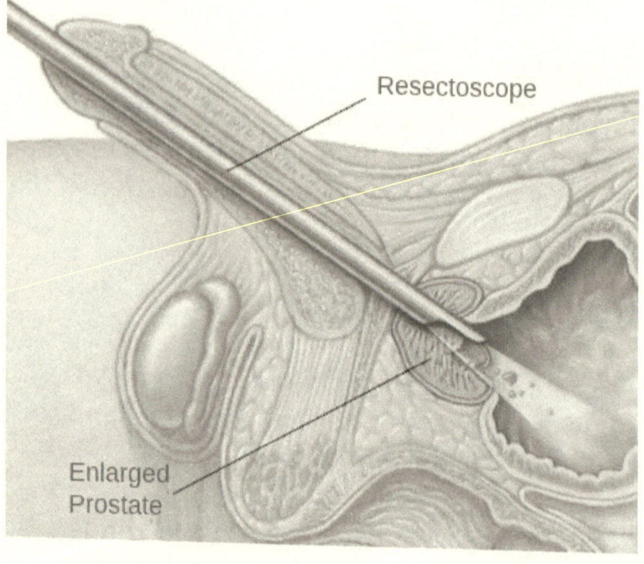

A long, thin instrument with a camera is inserted up the urethra to reach your prostate, where the enlarged tissues are removed using an electrical loop.

     Quality Solutions

The loop not only cuts, but also cauterizes the blood vessels to control bleeding.

Another type of surgery is the **TUIP** (transurethral incision of the prostate) procedure.

TUIP widens the urethra to allow for stronger urine flow.

Open surgery requires an external incision to reach the prostate. This procedure is only used under more severe circumstances.

Prostate artery embolisation
The aim of this procedure is to reduce the blood supply of the prostate gland, causing some of it to die off with subsequent shrinkage. Embolisation involves the introduction of micro particles to block these small prostatic arteries. Embolisation agents include polyvinyl alcohol (PVA), gelatin sponge and other synthetic biocompatible materials.

Laser surgery
A thin laser fibre is positioned within the laserscope and is passed up through the urethra to deliver the treatment. Patients are usually able to return home on the same day.

Lifestyle

Lifestyle does influence to a degree the development of BHP and can assist in reducing growth.

As mentioned earlier, being overweight puts you at a disadvantage.

However men who are physically active are less likely to suffer from BPH. Even low- to moderate-intensity physical activity, such as walking regularly at a moderate pace, yielded benefits.

The message really is stay active.

Diet

Whilst we should not cut down on the amount of water we drink, we don't want to pee more often than necessary.

Now, there are some foods which exacerbate the need to pee so if we reduce the amount of those then it will to an extent ease the situation.

These are the natural diuretics, meaning they increase and encourage urine production.

These are:

Watermelon (one of the 'very best' diuretic fruits)
Pears
Peaches
Apples
Grapefruit
Grapes
Melon
Bananas
Cucumbers
Lettuce
Beets
Carrots
Brussels sprouts
Cabbage
Also cut down or eliminate the following:
Red meat
Eggs
Poultry
Spicy foods
Processed foods
Sugar
Sodium

Now I am not suggesting you give up eating all of these.

However have a look down the list and see if there are some you regularly eat in large quantities.
Try doing without them for a few weeks and see if anything changes.

On the other side of the coin, here are some foods that may help reduce the problems of an enlarged prostate.

Fish,
Especially salmon, herring, sardines, anchovies and Trout.
Berries,
like strawberries, blackberries, and raspberries.
Vegetables,
Green leafy vegetables, broccoli, cauliflower.
Salad items,
like bell peppers, tomatoes, avocados
Nuts,
Brazil, pecans,almonds, and walnuts.
Seeds,
Sesame, pumpkin, ground flax.
Olive oil
Garlic, onions, shallots, leeks and chives.

Health Bites

Health Bites are deliberately very short books.

They cover just one specific health issue and all offer solutions or ways to reduce the problem.

In them I give the whys, wherefores and practical help in resolving health issues.

Positive suggestions that are aimed at curing the issue is the philosophy behind all of these guides.

This guide is on the Prostate Gland and hones in on how to start reducing the problem from today onwards.

Prostate is just one of a series of short to the point guides on health matters that are relevant to our lifestyles.

Disclaimer

I am not a doctor, please check with your medical practitioner before following any health advise given in this e-book or elsewhere.

The materials in this e-book are provided "as is" and without warranties of any kind either

express or implied.
The Author disclaims all warranties, express or implied, including, but not limited to, implied warranties of merchantability and fitness for a particular purpose.

Under no circumstances, including, but not limited to, negligence, shall the Author be liable for any special or consequential damages that result from the use of, or the inability to use this e-book, even if the Author or his authorized representative has been advised of the possibility of such damages. Applicable law may not allow the limitation or exclusion of liability or incidental or consequential damages, so the above limitation or exclusion may not apply to you. In no event shall the Author's total liability to you for all damages, losses, and causes of action (whether in contract, tort, including but not limited to, negligence or otherwise) exceed the amount paid by you, if any, for this book. Facts and information are believed to be accurate at the time they were placed in this book. All data provided in this e-book is to be used for information purposes only. The information contained within is not intended to provide specific medical, legal, financial or tax advice, or any other advice whatsoever, for any individual or company and should not be relied upon in that regard. The services described are only offered in jurisdictions where they may be legally offered.

Information provided is not all-inclusive, and is limited to information that is made available and such information should not be relied upon as all-inclusive or accurate.

This and all the other Health Bites are short guides for a possible quick fix solution. They are not substitutes for consultations with your doctor.

I do hope this has helped you.

Feedback
Does it annoy you when there is no feedback on a product?

Help solve this by leaving feedback if you liked this.
But if you think this could be improve, please tell me so that I can improve it.
Thanks

Email me and let me know of any other subject I should research and publish.

Acknowledgements
NHS
Age UK
Mayo Clinic
Healthline

<u>Patient.co.uk</u>
<u>Harvard Medical School</u>
Illustration, Merck Manual Home Health Handbook, edited by Robert Porter. Copyright (2015) by Merck Sharp & Dohme Corp., a subsidiary of Merck & Co, Inc, Whitehouse Station, NJ. Available at <u>http://www.merckmanuals.com/home/</u>. Accessed (Jan 2015).

More information

My other books and ebooks all available on Amazon include:

Incontinence (part of Health Bite series)
Stress & anxiety solutions
Speak in Public ~ with ease, style & confidence
Remember anything ~ the easy way
My life changing journal
Bell-ringers' dots
Dots – just dots

Details of these and others can be found on Amazon by simply typing in John Harriyott

Please email me with suggestions for further Health Bites or your comments on this one, or anything else to <u>qualityman@quality-solutions.co.uk</u>

Charts

I have included some daily and weekly charts so that you can progress your improvements.

On the daily one just fill in a square every time you go. Start a new column each day then you will gradually build up a picture of your progress (or lack of).

Transfer the results onto the weekly chart as time passes.

This will help you and your doctor evaluate your progress.

I suggest you use a pencil for the chart. Then you can erase the results and re-use the page if needed.

Quality Solutions

S M T W T F S S M T W T F S S M T W T F S S M T W T F S S M T W T F S S M T W T F S S M T W T F S S M T W T F S

30
29
28
27
26
25
24
23
22
21
20
19
18
17
16
15
14
13
12
11
10
9
8
7
6
5
4
3
2
1
0

weeks

1 2 3 4 5 6 7 8 9 10 11 12 13 14 15 16 17 18 19 20 21 22 23 24 25 26 27 28 29 30 31 32 33 34 35 36 37 38 39 40 41 42 43 44 45 46 47 48 49 50 51 52

5 10 15 20 25 30 35 40 45 50 55 60 65 70 75 80 85 90 95 100 105 110 115 120 125 130 135 140 145 150

Quality Solutions

Weeks